THE LITTLE PINKY NO DRINKY BOOK

YOUR GUIDE TO MORE JOY AND HAPPIER
HOURS

CG FORD

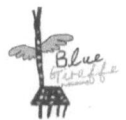

CONTENTS

EXCERPT: YOUR BEAUTIFUL
MIND: CONTROL ALCOHOL

This book is dedicated to Vincent Van Gogh, and other sensitive souls who want help to breakup with alcohol.
"I live soberly because I have a chance to do it, I drank in the past because I did not quite know how to do otherwise."
Vincent Van Gogh

INTRODUCTION

Many people drink too much and don't realise the harm they can cause themselves and others. Some know they have a problem and want to quit but don't know how to stop.

The Little Pinky No Drinky Book offers short sound bites of stand-alone readings designed to help you cultivate awareness and re-examine your relationship with alcohol amid the challenges of daily living.

This little book of big ideas offers a progressive programme of holistic—mental, emotional, physical and spiritual—support, guiding you through essential concepts, themes, and practices on the path to sobriety, well-being, joy, and happiness.

The tone is not preachy or moralising but wise, fun and joyful, with teachings presented in such a way that you'll say: "I get it. I understand. There is another way." Then, when the booze barons try to tempt you again, you'll see through their ruse and no longer be tempted to imbibe their toxic drugs.

Empowering and affirming quotes in each chapter by sober celebs will cheerlead you on and remind you you're not alone.

All that I share are strategies that have worked for me personally through many of my own life challenges and for my clients in my professional work as a holistic therapist, joyologist and self-empowerment coach.

A central tenet of this book is to provide you with information and education that counteracts the dominant messages provided by booze barons whose purpose in life is to help you drink more. Of course, they want you to drink—their mission is to spin a grand profit. I also aim to share with you simple and powerful well-being strategies you can apply yourself—many from the comfort of your own home.

What you're about to discover may be eye-opening, mind-changing or rejuvenating reinforcement to follow through on what you already know. The end goal? To make informed choices about what you are ingesting, how much, and why—and to be empowered to change your relationship with alcohol once and forever.

How to Benefit From This Book

Turn to a page at random or read this book sequentially, and return to it again and again when you need a pep talk.

I offer this book with love and hope this book is helpful to you.

P.S. Read to the end for a bonus excerpt: *Mind Your Drink: Control Alcohol and Love Your Life More.*

1

WHY DO YOU DRINK?

Why do you drink? To belong? To numb your feelings? Distract yourself? Reduce the pain or unhealed trauma?

Who would you be if you didn't drink? The outsider? The loser? The loner? Or the cool person who's naturally high?

"I didn't realise that I was an alcoholic until I realised that the alcohol was not for fun anymore. It was medicine."

Alice Cooper

2
_____

WHY DO YOU WANT TO QUIT

W anting to break up with alcohol doesn't make you an alcoholic. There are many reasons for stopping. Increasingly popular motivations include:

- Losing weight
- Gaining more time
- Increasing success
- Fulfilling your potential
- Having money
- Being in control of your mind, body and soul
- More joy and longer happier hours
- Saving your life
- Freedom!

WHY DO you want to quit?

"Drinking worked in the beginning: I felt wonderful, warm, and fuzzy… almost pretty…What I didn't know was that I was in a prison of my own making."

Colette Baron-Reid

3

WHAT'S WRONG?

I dentify what's wrong to stay strong. Is alcohol draining your motivation and energy? Ruining your sleep? Destroying your mental and spiritual health? Or something else?

Take a negative and make a positive—quit.

"I gave up alcohol in 1980. I enjoyed it far too much, so I frequently got intoxicated. Everything in my life changed for the better when I stopped. It was the right decision."

Deepak Chopra

4

WHAT'S YOUR POISON?

Alcohol is ethanol masquerading as a happy drink. It's a toxic, psychoactive, highly addictive, dependence-producing substance that causes a host of both mental and physical illnesses, including cancer.

The International Agency for Research on Cancer has classified alcohol as a Group 1 carcinogen. This is the highest-risk group, including asbestos, radiation, and tobacco. Recent alerts by Public Health authorities warn there is no safe level of alcohol consumption in terms of preventing a number of illnesses.

"Then you shall know the truth, and the truth will set you free."

John 8:32

PAIN OR PLEASURE?

Life is a combination of two things: running away from pain and running towards pleasure. Booze bridges both impulses.

Break the circuit switch to a pleasurable passion. Enjoy a happier, healthier high.

"I was so concerned what you thought of me, how I was coming across, how I would survive the day. I always felt like an outsider. I just lived in my head. I realised I wasn't going to live up to my potential, and that scared the hell out of me."

Bradley Cooper

ALCOHOL IS A DRUG

Alcohol is a highly addictive, readily available, mind-altering legalised drug. Within 90 seconds, the ethanol in alcohol will affect all the organs and systems in your body, crossing even the blood-brain barrier, which usually keeps harmful substances away from the brain.

It affects the brain's prefrontal cortex, responsible for decision-making and rational thinking. Under the influence of alcohol, people are likely to make impulsive decisions without considering the consequences. It can also induce psychosis in some people.

"It's a hell of a drug, man."

Dr Jordan Peterson

DOWNERS AND UPPERS

I t doesn't matter how high you felt drinking booze the night before. Alcohol is a downer. It depresses your central nervous system, spikes anxiety and makes you feel low. Find a happy, healthy high that keeps on giving naturally.

"I finally summoned up the courage to say three words that would change my life: 'I need help.' Thank you to all the selfless people who have helped me on my journey through sobriety. I am eternally grateful."

Elton John

WEIGHT WOES

A lcohol packs a weight of sugar. It makes booze taste sweeter and increases its addictive load. No wonder you find it hard to say 'no' and pile on the fat. The truth is you're slimmer and sexier sober.

"Extremes are to be avoided."

Leonardo da Vinci

WHO INSPIRES YOU?

Some of the coolest, most successful people on the planet don't drink. Drew Barrymore, Colin Farrell, Tom Hardy, Eric Clapton, Russell Brand, Brene Brown, Blake Lively, Ewan McGregor, J-Lo, Bradley Cooper, Lilly Allen, Dr Jordan Peterson and Brad Pitt are just a few.

Fun, healthy, thriving people gave up booze. Will you?

"I have yet to meet a person whose sobriety has made their life worse. I have yet to—but I am open to it. If you find someone, please get in touch with me because I would love to have a chat with them and ask them a couple of questions. I have yet to meet a person whose sobriety didn't make a better father, a better friend."

Colin Farrell

FINANCIAL RESCUE

Quitting drinking does magical things for your savings, career and health. Drinking is expensive, compromises your judgement and often leads to poor decisions. Many people's finances are financially rescued when they give up booze. Let that be you.

"Staying sober really was the most important thing in my life now and had given me direction when I thought I had none."

Eric Clapton

THE DAILY HABIT

Take sobriety day by day. Just for today, decide not to drink.

"When I started, I took it one day at a time. Ultimately, I found that spirituality worked for me."

Russel Brand

THINK NO DRINK!

Your thoughts create your reality. Think 'sexier, saner, successful sober without that drink!'

"The problem of alcohol is, it's just too easy. It's everywhere. At least with hard drugs, you have to have a dealer. All I know is I could feel its presence in an ominous, daunting way that was preventing me from being my higher self."

Ben Harper

13

SWITCH!

Have you got the itch? Switch! Your mind can only focus on one thing. Distract yourself with something delightful.

"If you can't be available for the basic necessity of being there for your children, then something really needs to shift. It was that next day that I said, 'All right. It's time. Let's give this a shot.' And then a month went by, a couple of months went by, I'm [like], 'Alright. This feels good. This feels good.'"

Charlie Sheen

THE ART OF SOBRIETY

Allow yourself to acknowledge all that you feel without restraint. Paint, sing, write music, play an instrument —anything! Expressing yourself creatively will help you balance and heal your emotions.

"The crowd I was hanging with drank like world champions, and it slowly began to take over. Being that fucked up was not part of the dream. I wanted to play rock music, not be a junkie or alcoholic."

Duff McKagan

15

MAKE JOY FROM SH*T

When we show up for what we love, we can make magic from sh*t!

"I made a commitment to completely cut out drinking and anything that might hamper me from getting my mind and body together. And the floodgates of goodness have opened upon me spiritually and financially."

Denzel Washington

16

MOVE!

Exercise promotes the production of positive endorphins. These feel-good neuro-chemicals are vital in making you feel happier without leaning on alcohol.

Cycling, running, walking, and swimming are just a few ways to help beat the booze.

"I had a rusty old mountain bike in the garage and started riding. Ukidokan is also a big part of my everyday headspace. That became a new addiction."

Duff McKagan

FULL STOP!

E nough is enough! Give up drinking to excess. Inspire yourself to get sober.

"If I had woken up feeling pretty much fine, I probably wouldn't have been driven to rethink my whole life. But I was like, 'Oh, my God, I drink all the time."

Erin St-Pierre

STEP INTO YOUR POWER!

T ransform your addiction into something purposeful and beautiful.

"As time goes on, you turn into a puppet of your accumulated past. The lives of many people, for instance, are dominated by food or substance abuse. The primary problem is that they have set up a recurrent pattern in their life. But this software is not a fate to be endured. It can be rewritten, dropped, or distanced."

Sadhuguru

GO GRATITUDE!

G ratefulness for the blessings you have in life will lift you higher and higher.

"I didn't put (a drink) down because my drinking was a problem; I put it down because the way I drink leads me to have hangovers and those were the problem. My last hangover lasted for five days. It's irritating how well not drinking is going!"

Anne Hathaway

HAPPY HABITS

Set new intentions. What habits do you want to break? What happy habits do you want to create?

"I never really had a desire to do anything except get absolutely out of my mind. I loved it, but it's too painful on the body. After a while, you can't take it. I got to the point where I couldn't not get a hangover. And then, before you know where you are, it's taken five days to recover, and you're feeling terrible if you're not drinking, and it becomes a mess."

Damien Hirst

HEAL YOURSELF WITH WRITING

Create a bespoke journal tailored to support your sobriety needs. Include empowering quotes, inspirational people and recovery tips. Record your struggles and successes daily.

"Alcohol wasn't adding anything to my life. Sobriety delivers everything alcohol promised."

Drew Barrymore

ODE TO JOY

K ick the artificial highs and drunk delirium. Authentic joy delivers phenomenal happiness. Find joy in whatever is present in your life today.

"Hitting rock bottom and turning to my wife Faith Hill for support helped me get to the place I am today."

Tim McGraw

SAVE YOUR SOUL

When you're full of drink, an ugly statue sits where your soul should be. Spiritual practices will lift you into the realm of the 5th Dimension. Bath in the waters of spiritual healing. Meditate, pray, commune with nature or something else that soothes your soul.

"When I cut out alcohol, my life got better. When I cut out alcohol, my spirit came back. An evolved life requires balance. Sometimes, you have to cut one thing to find balance everywhere else."

Sarah Hepola

COSMIC CONSCIOUSNESS

E levate your consciousness and transcendent awareness. Raise your energy to 5D with sobriety.
The 5th dimension is...

- Pure love
- Pure light
- Unconditional forgiveness
- Unconditional awareness
- Instant manifestation
- Unlimited possibilities
- Beyond time and space
- The God vibration
- Expansion
- Healing
- Ascension
- Oneness
- Interconnectedness
- and so much more. . .

"We are all multidimensional beings with the potential to access higher Dimensions— higher states of consciousness— and because of this, we can heal ourselves faster now than ever before."

Kimberly Meredith

HAPPIER HOURS

P romising all the fun of booze in the sun without all the health hazards, alcohol-free concoctions are all the rage. Mix your own cool blends or buy AF off the shelf. Don't forget to use a lovely glass!

"*I* have some massive regrets for the mistakes I made when I was drinking. Some were deeply serious. Drink used to sustain me, but now I'm free."

Tracey Emin

PARTY SOBER

Are you feeling pressured to drink? Head for places that make sobriety fun. Arm yourself with your go-to-sobriety drink.

Prep yourself with a few good lines to say to people who try to encourage you to drink if your choices are challenged. For example:

"Alcohol makes me sick."

"I broke up with alcohol."

"I'm allergic to alcohol."

"I'm on a break."

Or something else that resonates with you.

"All the cool people I know are really into not drinking or are drinking a lot less."

Caitlin Walsh Miller

AFFIRM!

A ffirm the changes you want to see and be. Create and customise affirmations to support your intentions and empower with love-infused feelings. For example:

"I love getting drunk on painting and writing and creating abundance from my joy."

"I love being teetotal like successful people I admire."

"We are all born with gifts. Some of us have more than one.
What I do best is singing and dancing. But I never thought, as
I was correcting my life, that I would be recognised for it.
And my achievement is what I achieved after all of that ugly
life. How I achieved it was that my mind was clear.
No drugs. No alcohol."

Tina Turner

BEAUTY SLEEP

Alcohol plays havoc with sleeping patterns. Rediscover the joy of a good night's rest and be at your brilliant best. They don't call it 'beauty sleep' for nothing.

"Find happiness, health and financial freedom—drink more water!"

Sean Alexander

CELEBRATE!

G et a bottle of neurotoxins to celebrate? Why would you? Imbibe something deliciously extraordinary instead. Your favourite food? A massage? A pedicure? A new book? The list is endless.

"Getting sober remains my single greatest accomplishment."

Jamie Lee Curtis

YOU ARE NOT ALONE

F eel supported. Find the people who think and feel like you do.

"We can talk ourselves into death, or we can talk ourselves into the best life we've ever lived. So wherever you are, get help. Don't be ashamed. Be proud of yourself — whatever you do, don't let anyone put you down."

Sir Anthony Hopkins

BORED TO BRILLIANT

Many people drink so much booze that they are borderline alcoholics without knowing it. Often, boredom is the culprit. But what if the opposite was also true? What if, by quitting drinking, you could go from bored to brilliant by channelling your energies into doing something magnificent?

"I stopped drinking maybe like three and a half months ago. It's boring. I mean, I was literally borderline alcoholic for quite a lot of my 20s, but I miss it so much."
Adele

FILL THE VOID

This little book of big ideas in tiny little sound bites has shared a sweet suite of progressive, holistic tools—mental, emotional, physical and spiritual. We've explored many concepts, themes, and practices to help you find beautiful sobriety, well-being, joy, and happiness.

Some of the many supportive practices we've explored include: swamping a negative addiction for a positive obsession, expressing yourself creatively, finding and following your passion and purpose, meditating, journaling, joining a support group, reciting affirmations, and being inspired by other sober-cool people.

Whatever your motivation, you've discovered that you're not alone in the desire to quit the booze. Millions of people suffer the impact of alcohol harm. In the US alone, there are over 50 million children and adult children of alcoholics.

I want to reinforce maintaining sobriety on this drunk-crazed planet is not a given. Being a rebel with a sober cause takes daily devotion and dedication. But on this, everyone in recovery agrees: you're a better person, partner, friend, and creative spirit alcohol-free.

Removing alcohol won't leave a void. Just the opposite. You'll gain your self-worth and self-respect. You'll unlock the floodgates of your potential and open the doors for new dreams to be achieved. You'll give up one thing (booze) to have everything!

"I'm all alone, save for my good friends Johnnie Walker and Grey Goose. 'You've got everything,' I thought, 'but you've really got f——all. The huge hole, the void, I had to fill somehow. I filled it with booze. And it nearly killed me."
Phi Collins

FREE BONUS!

The Passion Journal: The Effortless Path to Manifesting Your Love, Life, and Career Goals

Thank you for your interest in my new book.
To show my appreciation, I'm excited to be giving you another book for FREE!

Download the free *Passion Journal Workbook* here>>https://dl.bookfunnel.com/aepj97k2n1

I hope you enjoy it—love is the new drug. This book is dedicated to helping you enjoy sobriety and to live and work with passion, resilience and joy.

You'll also be subscribed to my newsletter and receive free giveaways, insights into my writing life, new release advance alerts and inspirational tips to help you live and work with passion, joy, and prosperity. Opt out at anytime.

OTHER BOOKS YOU MAY ENJOY

Health & Happiness:

The Happy, Healthy Artist
Stress Less. Love Life More
*Bounce: Overcoming Adversity, Building Resilience and
Finding Joy*
Bounce Companion Workbook

Mindful Sobriety:

Mind Your Drink: The Surprising Joy of Sobriety
*Mind Over Mojitos: How Moderating Your Drinking Can
Change Your Life: Easy Recipes for Happier Hours & a Joy-
Filled Life*
Your Beautiful Brain: Control Alcohol and Love Life More

Happy Sobriety:

Happy Sobriety: Non-Alcoholic Guilt-Free Drinks
You'll Love

The Sobriety Journal
Happy Sobriety Two Book Bundle-Box Set: Alcohol and
Guilt-Free Drinks You'll Love & The Sobriety Journal

EXCERPT: YOUR BEAUTIFUL MIND: CONTROL ALCOHOL

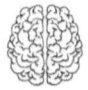

ABOUT THIS BOOK

Many people drink too much and don't realise the harm they can cause themselves and others. Some know they have a problem, but don't know how to solve it.

Alcohol misuse results in thousands of preventable deaths and hospitalisations every year from accidents, violence, and diseases including liver damage and cancer. The cost, in dollars alone, is truly staggering, estimated at billions per year. The price of heartache is incalculable. In New Zealand, and other Western cultures suicide is the leading cause of death, especially amongst our young people. Alcohol is a major contributing factor.

Alcohol, we are told, makes us happy. Very little is said about the side-effects—anxiety, depression, aggression.

Your Beautiful Mind: Control Alcohol & Love Life More provides an antidote by promoting a more mindful and responsible drinking culture.

It aims to help reverse the harm of alcohol. The goal is to normalise, not stigmatise sobriety. The agenda is to help you take back control, push back the booze barons' unbalanced and misleading ploys and restore the balance. The hope is that after reading this book, wellness will be the priority for all people regardless of circumstances and race.

It offers short, sound-bites of stand-alone readings designed to help you cultivate awareness and reexamine your relationship to alcohol amid the challenges of daily living.

Your Beautiful Mind: Control Alcohol & Love Life More offers a progressive program of holistic—mental, emotional, physical and spiritual—support, guiding you through essential concepts, themes, and practices on the path to sobriety, well-being, joy, and happiness.

The tone is gently humorous, sometimes challenging, occasionally provocative, but always compassionate and kind, and, I hope infinitely wise.

My aim is not to sound preachy or moralising, but to present information in such a way that you'll say: "I get it. I understand. There is another way." And then, when the booze barons try to tempt you again, you'll see through their ruse and no longer be tempted to imbibe their drugs.

All that I share are strategies that have worked for me personally through many of my own life challenges, and for my clients in my professional work as a holistic psychologist and self-empowerment coach.

A central tenet of this book is to provide you with information and education that counteracts the dominant messages provided by booze barons whose purpose in life is to help you drink more. Of course, they want you to drink—their mission is to spin a grand profit. I also aim to share with you simple and powerful well-being strategies you can apply yourself— many from the comfort of your own home.

What you're about to discover may be eye-opening, mind-changing or rejuvenating reinforcement to follow through on what you already know.

The end goal? To make informed choices about what you

are ingesting (ethanol and sugar), how much, and why—and to be empowered to change your relationship with alcohol once and forever.

Armed with the truth about alcohol you will gain:

- A new way to see and understand your relationship to alcohol
- The removal of the fear and stigma of admitting you need help
- Insight into the reasons why drinking too much is not your fault and that you have just become another cultural conditioning statistic
- Simple strategies to take back control

Your Beautiful Mind: Control Alcohol & Love Life More will strengthen your subconscious desire NOT to drink and help you make healthy, lasting, self-empowered change.

Experts suggest that it takes months, even years, of hardship to stop drinking. This book challenges this diagnosis and offers a different solution—and works...fast.

But at the end of the day, no one can make you control your drinking. You have to want to change. It is my hope that *Your Beautiful Mind* will strengthen your intention to quit or cut back drinking. The choice is yours, my friend.

Within this choice, is the chance to seek help, or not, for problems that keep you stuck, peer pressure that keeps you drinking, or traumas and open wounds that need healing—not numbing with alcohol.

I hope you will choose to free yourself from pain so that you may find the freedom, happiness, health, and joy you deserve and which awaits.

Your Beautiful Mind features the most essential and stirring passages from some of my previous books, exploring topics such as meditation, mindfulness, positive health behaviours, and touches on ways to working with fear, depression, anxiety, and other painful emotions.

Your Beautiful Mind: Control Alcohol & Love Life More expands upon these previous books and blends the latest scientific research, spotlights the cultural, social, and industry factors that support alcohol dependence, and also encourages a more holistic and mindful approach to the seriousness of life and the ever-present stressors we all face.

As one advance reviewer wrote to me before reading *Your Beautiful Mind*, "The people who I work with are wanting to eliminate alcohol from their lives and rebuild their lives, families, and relationships. They do not want permission, approval or instruction on how to drink mindfully."

However, after reading this book, he wrote, "I really like the approach that this book takes in not attempting to stop drinking totally. It instead explains and coaches how to manage and cope with consuming alcohol so that the damaging effects may be minimised. This is a very useful supportive book for 'drinkers' and their families."

The purpose of this book is not to trivialise, nor condone, legitimise, or sanction problem drinking. Being mindful doesn't mean being obstinately blind to the very real perils of alcohol abuse and addiction.

Being mindful is a call to awakening and purposeful action to build the life you want—free of addiction.

It's a willingness to consider the growing evidence that shows there is a different way—a lasting and empowering solution, and it's one you can master yourself.

Through the course of this book, you will learn practical, creative and simple methods for overcoming subconscious scripts that keep you craving alcohol, heightening awareness and overcoming habitual patterns and addictive behaviours that block happiness and joy and hold you back.

Brimming with a smorgasbord of easy-to-apply strategies that will boost your mental, emotional and physical well-being, *Your Beautiful Mind: Control Alcohol & Love Life More* is a timeless call to action for anyone who wants to cut back or quit drinking alcohol, get their life back and create a healthier, happier, joyful time on this planet.

Three Holistic Principles of Success

Your Beautiful Mind takes a holistic look at what it means, and what it takes, to control alcohol. Everything is interconnected: mind, body, and spirit. To succeed in your quest to control alcohol you'll need to unify and empower them all.

To avoid overwhelm and facilitate a selection of healing options I've sectioned *Your Beautiful Mind* into a cluster of principles. Principles aren't constricting rules unable to be shaped, but general and fundamental truths which may be used to help guide your choices.

Let's look briefly at The Three Principles of Sobriety and what each will cover:

Principle One, "The Call for Sobriety" will help you explore the truth about controlling alcohol and define sobriety on your own terms. You'll discover the rewards and 'realities' of becoming booze free, and intensify success-building beliefs. You may realise you have a problem, but many people don't. In this section, we'll look at definitions of what constitutes problem drinking—and what doesn't. We'll also explore the reasons you drink, the biology of emotions and how to get naturally high.

You'll learn some truths which powerful business would

rather see hidden and clarify the huge costs alcohol imposes on all of us in **Principle Two, "Rethinking Drinking."** You'll also discover why love, anger, igniting the fire within, and heeding the call for self-empowerment is the cornerstone of future success.

Actions shout louder than words. **Principle Three: "Strategies for Sobriety,"** will help you take back control. You'll learn how to tame your subconscious mind, deal with stress, trauma, societal pressure, and other life-stuff that may drive you to drink.

Love will be your new drug of choice. Love for yourself, your significant others, and your life. Passion, purpose, joy—call it what you will—love is the cure for all our ills.

It sounds simple. And it is.

In this section of the book, you'll clarify and visualise what you really want to achieve. You'll then be better able to decide where best to invest your time and energy. You'll also begin exploring ways to develop your life and career in light of your passions and purposeful sobriety, maintain focus and bring your vision to successful reality.

Strategies to help you empower your spirit urge you to pay attention to the things that: feed your soul; awaken your curiosity; stir your imagination; and create passion in your life. You'll also discover how to strengthen your connection to your superconscious mind.

You may be surprised to discover that you have three minds, and more—you'll discover ways to empower them all to overcome obstacles, achieve greater balance and fulfilment and maximise your sobriety success.

Your health is your wealth yet it's often a neglected part of success. Techniques to help you heal and empower your body recognise the importance of a strong, flexible and healthy body to your mental, emotional, physical and spiritual success.

You'll be reminded of simple strategies which reinforce the importance of quality of breath, movement, nutrition, and sleep.

Avoiding burnout is also a huge factor in maintaining sobriety. When you do less and look after yourself more, you can and will achieve freedom from alcohol.

Throughout Your Beautiful Mind, you'll also boost your awareness of how surrounding yourself with your vibe tribe will fast-track your success, and when it's best to ditch your booze buddies or go it alone.

Even if you think you've got the alcohol thing licked or you don't believe you're addicted, find a sprinkling of inspiring people and discover their successful strategies to control their drinking or to quit.

Discovering some of the most successful ways people have overcome their dependence on alcohol or addiction to booze and achieved freedom for good will boost your belief in the fact that it's easy, simple, and within your control.

Where there's a will—there is a way.

You'll be inspired by others success. Importantly you'll learn how following your own truth will set you free.

HOW TO USE THIS BOOK

If you've been drinking too much, or just getting in your own way, you're in good company, many successful, talented, beautiful people have been there. I've been there too. Guess what, drinking too much and getting in your own way is, sadly, normal.

I promise there are solutions to the problems you're currently facing—and you'll find them in the pages that follow.

Dig into this book and let me, and other alcohol control experts, be your mentor, inspiration and guide as we call forth your passions, purpose, and potential.

Through the teachings of others, extensive research into alcohol recovery, the biology of desire and neurology of addiction and the mysteries of motivation, success, and fulfilment, *Your Beautiful Mind: Control Alcohol & Love Life More* will help you accelerate success.

Plus, I'll share a candid peek at my own personal experience, including many unsuccessful efforts to scale back my drinking—and how I found a strategy that was fun, fabulous and worked.

You'll also benefit from my experience and professional success with clients as a holistic therapist.

Together, we will guide you to where you need to go next and give you practical steps to control alcohol and find freedom and happiness.

Growing up I wasn't encouraged to drink less. My hope is that after reading *Your Beautiful Mind: Control Alcohol & Love Life More,* you will be!

Step into this ride joyfully and start creating your best life today.

• If you want to have more energy and fire in your belly

• If you want to have happy, healthy, loving relationships

• If you want to stress less and love life more

• If you want to improve your mental, emotional, physical and spiritual health...

Then *Your Beautiful Mind: Control Alcohol & Love Life More* is exactly the right the book for you—whoever you are, whatever challenges you are facing and however you define health, happiness, and sobriety.

The ideas described in this book apply to anyone who's trying to control alcohol and inject some purposeful sobriety into their life and work.

Your Concise Guide to Success

Your Beautiful Mind: Control Alcohol & Love Life More is a concise guide to controlling alcohol. My vision, like many of my other self-empowerment books, was simple: a few short, easy to digest tips for time-challenged, distraction-loaded, people who were looking for inspiration and practical strategies to encourage positive change.

In this era of information overload and distraction, I knew

that people didn't need a large wad of words to feel inspired, gain clarity and be stimulated to take action.

In coaching and counselling sessions I'd encourage my clients to ask a question they would like answered. The questions could be specific, such as, 'How can I stop drinking?' Or vague, for example, 'What do I most need to know?' They were always amazed at how readily answers flowed.

The need for simple, life-affirming messages is so important. If you are looking for inspiration and practical tips, in short, sweet sound bites, this guide is for you.

Similarly, if you're a grazer, or someone more methodical, this guide will also work for you. Pick a section or page at random, or work through the tips sequentially. I encourage you to experiment, be open-minded and try new things. I promise you will achieve outstanding results.

Let experience be your teacher. Give your brain a well-needed break. Balance 'why' with how you feel and embrace how you feel or how you want to feel. Honour the messages from your intuition and follow your path with heart.

At the time of writing, I've just turned to the chapter, *Your Body Barometer*. It's a timely reminder that when you drink too much your mental, emotional and spiritual health can suffer.

The following remark from Coco Chanel may also speak to you: "I invented my life by taking for granted that everything I did not like would have an opposite, which I would like."

Your Caffeine Hit

As with my other wellness books, I encourage you to Think of *Your Beautiful Mind: Control Alcohol & Love Life More* as a shot of espresso. Sometimes one quick hit is all it takes to energise your willpower, improve your mood, or kickstart your resolve.

But sometimes you need a few shots to sustain your energy. Or maybe you need a bigger motivational hit and then you're on your way.

You're in control of what you need and what works best for you. Go at your own pace but resist over-caffeinating. A little bit of guidance here and there can do as much to fast-track your success as consuming all the principles in one hit.

Skim to sections that are most relevant to you and return to familiar ground to reinforce home-truths. But most of all, exercise compassion and enjoy your experience.

DIVE DEEPER With *The Sobriety Journal: The Easy Way to Stop Drinking: The Effortless Path to Being Happy, Healthy and Motivated Without Alcohol*

Creating a Sobriety Journal was a major aid in my own recovery—you'll find some excerpts sprinkled throughout *Your Beautiful Mind: Control Alcohol,* and I've written a handy resource to help you create your own.

This guided book leaves you free to create your own bespoke journal tailored to support your needs. It includes, Journal Writing Prompts, Empowering and Inspirational Quotes and Recovery Exercises that can be of use in your daily journal writing, working with your sponsor or use in a recovery group.

AVAILABLE IN PRINT and eBook at all good online retailers.

YOUR BEAUTIFUL MIND Workbook

Your Beautiful Mind: Control Alcohol & Love Life More print book will also be available as a workbook, with space to write your responses to the challenges and calls to action within the book.

STRESS LESS, Love You More & Create a Beautiful, Successful LifeToday!

INTRODUCTION: THE TRUTH
ABOUT SOBRIETY

S obriety
     Noun

1. the state or quality of being sober
2. temperance or moderation, especially in the use of alcoholic beverages
3. seriousness, gravity, or solemnity

"I THOUGHT you were going to tell me I couldn't drink at all," said my partner when I mentioned the title of this book.

Nope, sobriety does NOT mean abstinence. Although, some organisations like Alcoholics Anonymous define it that way. However, for a great many people abstinence is truly the only path to freedom.

Whether you're flirting with the idea of sobriety or starting out on your sober journey, you'll be glad to hear that sobriety, however you define it is about living life on your terms.

Your Beautiful Mind is not about telling anyone how much to drink or not to drink—the focus is on helping you make more informed decisions and empowered choices.

And, I'll be honest, my hope is that after reading this book you'll truly feel liberated. Liberated from the myth that committing to sobriety sentences you to a grey wasteland of boredom, devoid of pleasure and plagued with seriousness.

In fact, as you'll find the exact opposite. Sobriety is sexy, empowering, fun and smart. And you don't have to take it from me. Ask Jennifer Lopez, Colin Farrell, Russell Brand— me, and a whole bunch of other people who know life truly is more beautiful sober.

The truth about alcohol is that sobriety and abstinence have been given a bad rap. But the tide is turning as more and more people grow disenchanted with booze and the addiction of despair.

"Sobriety" is a word whose 12-step misuse now pervades our entire culture, along with ruining addiction treatment," says addiction expert Dr. Stanton Peele.

"In fact, the DSM psychiatric manual (unbeknownst to virtually everyone who uses it, including even experts who write about it) says Peele, contains no abstinence criterion for recovery (actually called remission)."

Sobriety is more than being a tee-total. It's more than fighting a daily battle with your willpower. It's more than the number of drinks you do, or don't knock back.

Sobriety actually means not drinking alcohol in excess, being intoxicated, or drunk. In the true context being sober means not being pissed, sobbing into your wine, puking your guts out, being a dickhead, a violent vermin or lying comatose in a gutter somewhere.

Ultimately, whether you opt for abstinence or moderation,

controlling alcohol involves choice. The choice to drink, or not to drink.

"Yeah, right, you can control alcohol," a woman wrote in an alcohol forum when I shared the title of this book.

Granted, controlling alcohol, like controlling anything pervasive, takes concentrated, disciplined and motivated effort. Not only are you swimming against a tide of historical attitudes to alcohol that infect so many people today, but plenty of booze barons and associated industries gain eye-watering profits by persuasively encouraging you to drink more…and more…and more.

It seems as though everywhere you look somebody is trying to slip you another drink.

You're not even safe at home. The other day I received a delivery from BookDepository. Inside the package lay a bookmark advertising a staggering range of wines I could order online. And there I was thinking I had simply ordered a book. Nope, there is no escaping the onslaught.

But you can master the art of ignoring peoples' attempts to seduce you with their booze temptations and you can become a pro at zoning out.

It's incredibly liberating and empowering when armed with the truth about alcohol, you're no longer in its grip.

That's how it is for me, and it's how it can be for you. I started writing this book thinking I'd just scale back my drinking a weeny bit, but I discovered the life-changing magic of complete abstinence, not because I couldn't drink—but because I truly didn't want to.

And I'm betting that if you're willing to try my sobriety experiment you'll discover the surprising joy and life-changing benefits of abstinence.

Here are just a few:

- Better health
- More energy
- Greater enthusiasm for life
- Deeper and more fulfilling relationships
- Improved finances
- Deeper spiritual connection
- Enhanced creativity
- Elevated well-being,
- Peace of mind
- Freedom
- Happiness
- True joy
- Increased brainpower

....and so many more benefits we'll explore further in this book.

Be Empowered

Despite compelling evidence of both the considerable health risks of drinking alcohol, in many countries, including New Zealand, heavy or binge drinking, defined as having five or more drinks in one sitting at least once a month in the past year, has become the accepted norm.

Disturbingly, drinking to excess is actively encouraged as 'freedom of choice' and 'alcohol fuelled fun'.

Yes, you do have free choice. But if you're going to make better decisions, you'll need better information.

Interestingly, improving education is a tactic the New Zealand Police recently adopted. At least 30 underage drinkers, all aged between 14 and 17, were collared for breaching Wanaka's public liquor ban during the December 31 2017 public street party.

Instead of slapping them with a $250 instant fine, the police made them write essays about the impact of binge drinking on their teenage brains.

Worryingly, many said they got their alcohol from their parents—perhaps they too, should have been invited to put pen to paper. Increasing awareness is a key factor in changing any destructive habit.

Many people say they know they have a problem, they just don't know why they drink. We'll take a closer look at the diverse triggers that cause you to drink, why it's challenging to stop and how marketing moguls proactively feed your desire for their profitable vices.

The chapters in the section 'Rethinking Drinking' may be a sobering and timely reminder to cut back on the booze. You'll discover new knowledge, new choices, and discover how to get your fix from more positive addictions.

We'll also probe into the neurological causes of addiction. Once you understand the scientific, economic, cultural and systemic basis for your inexplicable behaviours and the truth about what alcohol does to your mind, body, soul, and relationships, you are unlikely to fall victim to addiction and alcohol abuse again. Even if it takes a few cycles of relapse to fully grasp the truth, you will be more empowered to fight back.

Best of all, once you've tasted life sober, mastered the art of living life raw, you'll be free. Life, even when crap happens, will be something you don't just survive, but joyfully, happily imbibe. You'll have mastered the art of living and the wisdom of no escape.

In the meantime, I encourage you to be a diagnostician —investigate alcohol in all its guises. Arm yourself with your own knowledge, don't just take it from me. And definitely, whatever you do, don't gain your knowledge from the booze barons. Seek impartial advice and be objective.

But first, let's test your knowledge. Then we'll take a look at the upside of drinking less. You'll be heartened to learn that quitting booze or reducing your daily quota is becoming cool. Sobriety, my friends, is the new drunk. You'll also discover, throughout this book, easy ways to get high naturally—swapping negative health-zapping addictions for positive life-affirming addictions—easily.

2

TEST YOUR KNOWLEDGE

"Drinking worked in the beginning: I felt wonderful, warm, and fuzzy... almost pretty...What I didn't know was that I was in a prison of my own making," says former addict Colette Baron-Reid—now a sober intuitive counsellor & author.

If you're worried about your drinking or have had a heavy drinking problem for a while chances are you're well aware of the signifiant health implications, and how alcohol ruins many areas of your life.

But many people aren't. They binge drink like it's a sport, scull drinks like there's no tomorrow. Ignoring the wake of devastation they leave in their path, they resist making a change for the better. Sometimes they leave it until it's too late to undo their mistakes.

If you feel that it's time to rethink the role and purpose of alcohol in your life. Test your current knowledge by answering the questions below:

- Do you know what alcohol really is?

- How is alcohol made? What process creates stronger spirits?
- Is alcohol a known cause for more than 60 different health conditions? Do you know what these are?
- Do you really understand the damage you're doing to your body when you're hung over?
- Why can a 5 percent beer can make you twice as drunk as a 4 percent version?
- What about an 8 percent craft beer? Is wine safer to drink than vodka?
- What is the definition of binge drinking? Can it kill you? Why can't you stop?
- Which country says it's fine to drink three pints a night?
- What is a unit of alcohol? What is a standard drink? Why does it matter?
- How many units of alcohol are deemed safe daily? Weekly? Why?
- Is it true that women should drink less than men?
- What are the health-effects and risk factors if you drink more than the recommended guidelines?
- Does alcohol depress the central nervous system at high doses?
- Did you know that alcohol can offer a short-term high, followed by deep lows, depression, anxiety and suicidal thoughts?
- Did you know that many alcoholic drinks include compounds called congeners that add to the taste, smell or colour of the drink? Why do they increase the likelihood and intensity of suffering a hangover, and other undesirable side effects?

- Do you really know what the labelling on the bottles you buy really means?
- Do you know that lobbyists influence governments so they can maximise the sale of alcohol to minors, and society's most vulnerable people?
- Do you even care? Are you happy remaining blissfully blind?

You'll find the answer to these questions in the pages that follow.

3

ALCOHOL UNMASKED

B ooze barons do such a great job of disguising alcohol that many people don't know what it really is.

Alcohol is ethanol, also known as ethyl alcohol or grain alcohol, and is a flammable, colourless chemical compound. Yes, folks, everything can really go up in flames when you drink.

I fondly remember Christmases spent at my grandmother's and the excitement we all felt when a match was held against the rum-soaked Christmas pudding and it burst into plumes of fire.

For some reason, until researching this chapter I never made the connection that booze was a flammable substance I poured down my throat.

Ethanol fuel is also used in some countries instead of gasoline in cars and other engines. In Brazil, for example, ethanol fuel made from sugar cane provides 18 percent of the country's fuel for cars.

In short, the alcohol or ethanol found in your favourite beer, wine, and spirits is a poison, masquerading as a happy drink. It's so toxic that, when consumed too quickly or in huge quantities, your body's default position is to expel it—usually in a totally unglamorous technicolor spray of vomit. That's if you're lucky.

Alcohol poisoning can, and does, cause death—both directly and indirectly through liver disease, breast cancer, and a staggering amount of other alcohol-related diseases. We'll explore the havoc caused by booze, as well as how sobriety leads to nirvana in the chapter, Health Havoc or Health Nirvana?

Yet, despite all the risks and dire health warnings, alcohol seems such a benign substance. Perhaps it's the allure of its origins—a uniquely natural process.

Alcohol is formed when oxygen deprived yeast ferments natural sugars found in fruits, grains, and other substances. For example, wine is made from the sugar in grapes, beer from the sugar in malted barley, cider from the sugar in apples, and most vodka from the sugar in fermented grains such as sorghum, corn, rice, rye or wheat (though you can also use potatoes, fruits or even just sugar.)

Many people use alcohol as a way to self-medicate their way through life's ups and downs. Peer into the history of alcohol and you'll find that its medical origins enjoy a good pedigree. Gin mixed with tonic containing quinine, for example, was historically used to treat malaria.

"So it's totally good for you," writes one enthusiastic supporter in an alcohol forum.

Yeah, if you've got malaria perhaps, but not if you're just sick and dog-tired of living.

Alcohol is classed as a 'sedative hypnotic' drug. That definition on its own may sound just like what you're craving until you discover the true impact. Sedative-hypnotic drugs depress the central nervous system (CNS) at high doses.

Hmmm, that doesn't sound so flash, especially if you're

prone to knocking back a few too many drinks. Your central nervous system controls a majority holding of the key functions of your body and mind. The CNS consists of two parts: your brain and your spinal cord.

As you know, the brain is the chief conductor of your thoughts, interpreting your external environment, and coordinating body movement and function, both consciously and unconsciously. Complex functions, including how you think and feel, and maintaining homeostasis, a relatively stable balance between all the interdependent elements in your body, are directly attributable to different parts of your brain.

Your spinal cord with its network of sensitive nerves acts as a conduit for signals between the brain and the rest of the body.

You definitely don't want to mess with the way this important duo functions. But every time you ingest alcohol you do, weakening their ability to perform like virtuosos, interfering with maintaining a healthy balance and the finely tuned harmony which is so vital to your health, performance and effectiveness, and causing all systems in your body to play horribly off key.

Would you love to possess an outstanding ability in your field? Excel in your chosen profession? Tap into higher knowledge? Hone a much-loved or admired skill? Be universally admired? Many people think alcohol aids the fulfilment of these desires—until they realise their beliefs were deceptively wrong.

Sobriety on the other hand... now there's a different story.

At lower doses, alcohol can act as a stimulant inducing feelings of euphoria, optimism, and gregariousness. Everything looks beautiful, your belief in yourself, your talents, and your ability elevates like a seductive piece of music. Your inhibitions float away, suddenly you imagine yourself to be far better than you really feel. Shyness disappears, in its place talkativeness.

For a little while.

But pour more and more drinks down your throat, knock back litres of your favourite elixir and you'll quickly find yourself confronted by the truth. Alcohol is trouble.

Quite simply, alcohol knocks the life out of you. The more you drink, the higher the likelihood you'll become drowsy. Recall the drunk in the corner, slouched against the wall, or the once vivacious life of the party, barely able to hold her head in her hands, as she sits slumped at the bar. I've been there—it's a predictable rite of passage. In a culture that values drinking, this is normal.

Normal but definitely not glamorous, hip or cool.

But things get worse. Sometimes much, worse. Your breathing naturally slows into a state called respiratory depression. It can become exceedingly shallow or worse, stop entirely—what's truly frightening is you have absolutely no control. No one chooses to fall into an alcohol-fuelled coma, but this is exactly what happens to far too many people.

Very high levels of alcohol in the body can shut down critical areas of the brain that control breathing, heart rate, and body temperature, resulting in death. And, tragically, far too many beautiful people needlessly die this way.

Can I scare you sober? It's not my agenda, but I do know this—that's exactly what happened to Amy Winehouse. And it's exactly what's happened to a great many other talented, beautiful, smart people. People who only wanted to feel high, but never intended to die.

As well as its acute and potentially lethal sedative effects at high doses, alcohol undermines every organ in the body and these effects depend on your blood alcohol concentration (BAC) over time.

We'll examine the dangers of drinking both large and small alcoholic beverages over a short period of time in the chapter, Binge Drinking Blindness.

We'll also dive deeper into what constitutes safe drinking, including analysing what constitutes a standard drink and why health authorities want you to control your drinking— assuming you don't want to kick the alcohol habit for good.

But first, let's stop to consider, how natural is alcohol really?

What's Hidden in Your Drink?

Ethanol made be created via a naturally occurring process, but that's not the end of the production cycle. The other thing to be mindful of is all the other hidden dangers lurking in your drinks.

Peer a little closer and you'll find all sorts of nasty additives—not to mention toxic sprays, pesticides, fungicides, chemical fertilisers and other things that infiltrate many crops. But you won't find many of these disclosed on the labels.

Sorry to spoil the party.

Health gurus cite dangerous levels of sulfites or sulphites (as it's spelled in New Zealand) and warn of harmful side-effects, particularly for those with a low tolerance.

The term sulphites is an inclusive term for sulphur dioxide (SO_2), a preservative that's widely used in wine-making (and most food industries) for its antioxidant and antibacterial properties. SO_2 plays an important role in preventing oxidisation and maintaining a wine's freshness.

When used in high levels, because it's considered harmful, it must legally be disclosed on product labels.

To be fair, many foods also contain sulphites. Some people claim the preservative is nothing to be alarmed by— unless of course, you include yourself in the numbers of people who are allergic. Sulphites cause bloating and itching in sulphite-sensitive people. Does your beloved have a beer gut or sulphite bloating?

Histamine High?

Some studies suggest sulphites and other additives, including compounds such as histamines and tannins, are connected to the pounding headaches many of us suffer after drinking. That, and our ballooning weight.

Fermented alcoholic beverages, especially wine, champagne, and beer are histamine-rich.

As the author and psychologist Doreen Virtue explains in her excellent book, *Don't Let Anything Dull Your Sparkle,* many people binge drink when stressed, but most don't realise that some of the excess weight may be attributed to stress-hormones and neurotransmitter responses. These biochemicals, Virtue says, are triggered by the fact when you're stressed you often binge on food and drinks to which you may unknowingly be allergic to, or which are intrinsically unhealthy.

As I've mentioned, any product that undergoes fermentation contains high levels of histamine. What I didn't know was that these histamines trigger allergic reactions in our body, especially if we're under a lot of stress.

Histamines get you both ways, not only occurring in the food and alcohol you drink, but also because when you're allergic to something your body releases its own histamine, says Virtue. "Stress produces histamine. We're all naturally allergic to stress," she says.

When you consume a diet that's high in histamine or histamine-inducing foods, your body becomes overwhelmed. Add a stressful lifestyle to the mix and it's no wonder you feel less than perky.

Histamines are also manufactured and released by our bodies not only when we're stressed but also when we're dehydrated. Again, alcohol, because it magnifies dehydration, makes things worse.

Virtue explains, "The trouble is that histamine produces uncomfortable symptoms such as bloating, itchy skin, profuse sweating, hot flashes, runny or stuffy nose, and feeling cold all the time, as well as low blood pressure, arrhythmia, anxiety, and depression."

Nice.

No wonder, we start to look and feel better when we lose the booze.

Other addictive beverages, like coffee and sugar-laden drinks also trigger histamine reactions. The net result is a 'histamine high.' This boosted energy and elation you experience is always short-lived and is always followed by an energy crash, plus other painful symptoms discussed above.

Before publishing her findings Virtue decided to test her theory and embark on a 30-day histamine-free diet.

"Within two days of going 'low-histamine,' I felt a youthful energy and exuberance that I had never experienced before. I felt well. I felt happy. And I knew it was due to the low-histamine diet... you cannot return to the old ways of bingeing upon histamine once you realize the process behind these binges."

Sugar Rush

Submerged in many alcoholic drinks are dangerous and highly addictive levels of sugar. Research collated in *New York Times* article stated, "Cravings induced by sugar are comparable to those induced by addictive drugs like cocaine and nicotine."

Latest research revealed in The New Zealand Listener in 2018 reveals the physiological and neurological reasons your brain makes you crave sugar. I share some of these findings in the chapter Sweet Misery. It's only since researching and writing this book that I realised I was more addicted to sugar than alcohol.

Whew! That's a relief. But it's also not—because both are tough habits to crack. Tough, but not impossible. Knowledge is power, right?

In summary, not only is alcohol a highly addictive poison, but your cravings, your weight gain, low energy levels and less-than-optimal mental and emotional health may be fuelled as much by additives and sugar, as it is ethanol or alcohol itself.

You can heal your life and it begins with examining the facts. Consider becoming an amateur sleuth and adopting the role of an investigative journalist. Discover how alcohol is made, including all the artificial things that are added to many products to make it tastier and more alluring—and potentially more dangerous to your health.

Perhaps this may be all the motivation you need to develop a healthy intolerance for alcohol.

4

SAVVY SOBRIETY

Many people struggle to control alcohol because they're not motivated by sobriety. But, being sober isn't just about not drinking.

Sobriety is achieved by putting energy and effort toward something you really desire.

Knowing *why* you want something is just as important as knowing *what* you want.

Why do you want to control your drinking? To feel better about your- self? To achieve wellbeing goals? Because you're afraid that your drinking it taking over your body and your life? To inspire others? Because you're curious that what you've been hearing is true—life really is better sober? Or something else?

We'll explore more ways to help you discover your driving purpose later in this book, but first here are just a few benefits of achieving sobriety:

- Improved mental health and wellbeing
- Better physical health

- Improved emotional health
- Elevated spiritual health
- Saves money
- Enriches your relationships
- Is an indispensable part of fulfilment
- Energises you
- Liberates you
- Will change your life and the lives of those who matter most to you

Being sober sounds great, and it is. But the challenge is that so many of us have been brainwashed into believing it's awesome to be drunk. As I share later in this book, many of the people we look up to, including our political leaders have a dysfunctional relationship with alcohol—no wonder it's hard to implement laws aimed at reducing alcohol harm.

But if it's cool to be high, why do so many of us want to quit? Why do thousands of people sign on for Dry July or make New Year's resolutions to lose the booze only to be coerced or bullied into drinking again?

Giving up drinking can feel like losing your best friend, even your lover—until you remind yourself how alcohol is a fickle companion who lets you down again and again.

Sobriety, now there's a forever friend.

She won't turn sour, she won't piss you off, or get mad at you, and she won't rob you blind. Sobriety won't hijack your brain and make you say and do things you'll wildly regret in the wake of hangover hell.

Sobriety is not seedy or unpleasant. Sobriety is a sophisti-cated, serene, stabiliser in a world gone mad.

Sober

Synonyms

1. Not drunk
2. Thoughtful, steady, down-to-earth and level-headed
3. Serene, earnest
4. Not addicted

Who doesn't want a friend like that?

Sadly, the opposite is also true. Some of my best, most trusted friends turn into tyrants, either at the time of drinking or in the days that follow. These are just a few of the changes I notice when they drink alcohol:

- Overly critical
- Short-tempered
- Tyrannical
- Moody
- Solemn
- Angry
- Silent
- Withdrawn

Here's a short excerpt from my Sobriety Journal:
29 Dec 2016.

"A terrible, terrible evening. Me hiding in fear. Brett on a rampage. Smashing my fridge (taking it physically out of the studio and hurling it to the ground). 'Stress' brought on by the windows he shattered when he mowed the lawn, his frustration at the fountain not going, mowing the front paddock and returning, his eyes flaming and puffy.

And then drinking. Three bottles of beer, then driving to

the store and returning with a giant bottle of Mount Gay rum which he knows I hate him drinking. It always makes him so aggressive. He drinks it straight from the bottle. I feel panic rising in my chest. I feel real fear. I fear for my life.

Smashed pots, plants, my canvases strewn with horrid words I cannot decipher.

*I'm cowering because I could quickly become a victim of his frenzied attack. I fear he has lost his mind. He **has** lost his mind. He has lost control.*

I really hate alcohol. I hate what it steals from me. Our love. Our dreams.

Although this frightening, truly terrorising episode happened so long ago, I still feel the fear. That's what traumatic episodes do to us—their linger in our body waiting to be triggered—or, with help, resolved. It's a chilling reminder, but also a motivating one, which fuels my commitment for sobriety, and my devotion to helping others free themselves from harm, save their relationships, regain their sanity—and so many of the other benefits sobriety promises and *delivers*.

Unlike alcohol, sobriety can be trusted.

Throughout this book I'll discuss some of my strategies for living in a booze soaked world, including how I keep my energy and vibration levels high and don't allow drunks to dull my sparkle.

One simple strategy I do find helpful, however, is to pin inspiring quotes somewhere visible to remind me to censure the tendency to demand others change or to judge.

Letting go of judgment creates peace, strength, and ultimately increases joy. Becoming judgment-free and leading by example is also one of the key sobriety steps recommended by many successful addiction programs. This includes self-judgment and self-criticism.

My current go-to quote is by Abraham Hicks, "Let others vibrate how they vibrate and want the best for them. Never mind how they're flowing to you. You concentrate on how you're flowing because one who is connected to the energy stream is more powerful, more influential than a million who are not."

You can see this quote, along with the image of a young woman in a glass jar, sending her loving light into the world. The jar represents the shield she places around herself, to protect her from negative people and dark outside forces.

I also invite love, not fear or anger to guide my day. I'm not saying it's easy—if it were the world would be a happier place. I work to remember how my loved ones are when they're sober—how kind they are, how caring. This love extends to me too. I know I'm a nicer, kinder person sober than I am drunk.

Exercising self-love, however, means accepting that sometimes there comes a time when being around people who abuse alcohol becomes too toxic. Their drinking may undermine your health, threaten your resolve, or cause you to constantly fear for your life. There are times you may have to quit not only the booze but people, places, and relationships that hold you back.

Finding joy in sobriety is a lifestyle choice—a very personal, and very empowered and empowering choice. It's a choice you make with eyes wide open, determined to celebrate and make the most of your one precious life in every way.

Humour, as you'll also discover, goes a long way.

This man is giving birth to a six-pack…'Father and beers are doing swell.'

It's a picture I drew in my Sobriety Journal, in part to remind me how staying sober improves my waistline.

Call it like it is....would you like a shot of ethanol and a gallon of sugar with that?

5

THE SURPRISING JOY OF SOBRIETY

I s it more fun to have one? The 'one-and-done' club is growing in popularity, despite considerable pressure to have more. Would you be happier? I know I am—'one or none', that's my new mantra. Rule number one, I never, ever drink when stressed.

Sobriety is my sunshine, my light, the sparkling clarity of a life infused with beauty. I love being sober. I love feeling in control.

Controlling alcohol has freed me from the darkness and despair that once stalked me, and which still haunts so many.

Sure, I no longer have the quick fix-magic potions to addle my brain, mask my fears, vanquish my insecurities. Making friends with social anxiety didn't come in a seductively beveled crystal flute fizzing with bubbles. Nope, it took a lot of hard graft.

But I have something more as a result. Heart-wide open I have my spirit, my soul, my self. I am supported, nourished, and free to be me—authentically, warts, vulnerabilities, flaws and all. And it feels great. And I never want to go back to the blindfolded darkness of short-term highs and long-term lows.

Self-love, self-compassion, self-acceptance, and self-care —they're all part of my toolkit. They're part of your toolkit too.

What do they all have in common?

Loving you.

Loving you more than trying to fit in with your drinking buddies. Respecting and loving your body and soul so much that you no longer crave toxins. Delighting in the fact you're riding a wave of new enlightened consciousness.

The World is Sobering Up

It's heartening to see the savvy sobers enjoying increasingly good company. Globally there's an awakening and with it a rebirth, a renaissance of sorts. Being boozed is a relic from the dark ages and this is the era of enlightenment. Sobriety is queen, abstinence her cohort.

Magazines are running pieces about the 'sober-curious' movement. *Elle* is printing headlines such as 'Why I Decided to Break Up With Alcohol'. Others are talking about how toxic and deadly alcohol is to your skin. *The Huffington Post* is running with 'What Alcohol Really Does to Your Sex Life', and *Men's Health* is asking 'Why Drinking a Little Booze Each Day May be Killing You'.

"I don't drink or smoke or have caffeine," music diva Jennifer Lopez was reported as saying, in a women's magazine. "That really wrecks your skin as you get older."

Yep, not only is sobriety for savvy connoisseurs of health and well-being, but being booze-free is becoming a status symbol.

Sober is the new drunk.

Think Colin Farrell, Russell Brand and Duff McKagan, bass guitarist of Guns N' Roses, and one of the world's greatest rock musicians. Sober and boring? I don't think so! Instead, they're admired, celebrated, held up as the new cool.

When I tell people I don't drink they look at me wide-eyed and full of awe. "Wow! I don't think I could function without a drink," many of them say. "I wish I could quit."

They can, you can—where there's a will, there is a way. Quite simply drinking alcohol is a habit, something many of us do without stopping to question why.

As the health risks become more and more apparent, and more valued, coupled with the unearthing of the tactical untruths peddled by suppliers, alcohol is going the way of cigarettes—on a fast-track trajectory out the door.

"I want to live. I don't want to die," UK songstress Adele famously declared when she shared her decision to considerably scale back her booze binging.

"I didn't want to live, but I didn't want to die," Colin Farrell once said before finding the courage and the will to quit drinking and seek help.

Your health is your wealth and sobriety will make you rich, a hundred times over. You'll find plenty of people investing in the new currency of sobriety.

Where once you couldn't party without a cigarette in your hand, or socialise without ingesting a plume of toxic smoke at a pub, booze-free bars, nightclubs and communities are sprouting like poppy seeds all around the world.

Having a Freaking Good Time Mindfully

"*No Beers, Who Cares* (BWC) isn't about making anyone feel bad about drinking. It's a movement towards shifting attitudes around how and why we drink and helping people become more aware of their beliefs and habits and having a freaking good time doing so," says Claire Robbie, the founder *No Beers, Who Cares*.

Robbie describes her *No Beers, Who Cares* initiative as not anti-alcohol, but as a pro-mindfulness initiative.

"There's a shift around the world as people understand how incredible life can be without drinking and it's time to bring that high vibration to New Zealand," Robbie says, "and it's an amazing step towards living more mindfully."

Claire Robbie was a news reporter on TV3's Nightline before a tumultuous time led her to discover the life-changing benefits of yoga and meditation and life without alcohol.

At a low point in her life, what started as a hobby became an essential part of her healing process, and as her love for her new practices grew, so did the awareness that she had discovered a new vocation.

"The focus is less about giving something up, but boosting your aware- ness of how much you gain," Robbie says.

Hack Your Habits Joyfully

"What we've seen is that giving up alcohol is a keystone habit. A keystone habit is one that unlocks your full well-being potential. Just a few of the benefits of going alcohol-free such as extra energy, motivation, vitality, productivity, money, and time, will begin to pave the way to the life you have always dreamed of," Robbie enthuses.

Whether you're tuning into *The Hello Sunday Morning* movement in Australia, *No Beers, Who Cares i*n New Zealand, *Morning Gloryville* or *Off The Rocks* in the UK, or the ever-growing number of bars that have taken alcohol out of the mix, you'll find safety in numbers.

"When I first decided to undergo a long-term sober stint

— total abstention from alcohol, for at least a few years and perhaps forever—I was full of dread, fear and feelings of deprivation, but after a while I realised how pivotal that decision was. It was only once I'd shelved alcohol that I was truly capable of sorting the rest of my life out. I then saw with absolute clarity how most people are addicted to something, and how the majority of those people are in denial about it," UK-based Jen Nelson, founder of Off The Rocks, says.

"I try not to waste time on regret, but if there's one thing I could go back and do differently, it would be to take a long and total break from alcohol a lot sooner than I did. Going sober for several years enabled me to identify the underlying causal reasons behind my once excessive drinking. Learning how to live sober also allowed me to cultivate proper coping techniques. I no longer celebrated every happiness with a drink and I stopped drowning my sorrows at the first sign of sadness. Recovery is so much more than giving something up, it's the way back to your authentic self."

How can you approach alcohol more mindfully? What might you be giving up by going alcohol free? How much might you gain? What are you prepared to change in your life? What would stop you?

Read on for further incentives on why sobriety is good for you, and why doing things to excess isn't just uncool but extremely dangerous—even fatal. Drink to excess, why would you? There comes a point in everyone's life when we decide, "I've had enough".

6

PROBLEM DRINKING?

"Not everyone who has a drinking problem will be able to see it," says recovering alcoholic and author of *Drink: The Intimate Relationship Between Women and Alcohol*, Anne Dowsett-Johnston.

Is your drinking already cause for concern? How do you know if you have a real problem, versus a temporary itch that you're using alcohol to scratch?

"If you want to know if you're getting into trouble, ask yourself ... are you drinking to numb? To numb feelings, to numb stress, to numb depression or anxiety?'" Dowsett Johnston says.

Alcohol makes us love life, we're told. If this is true, why aren't we a happier lot? Burnout, stress, anxiety have become worldwide epidemics—and with them alcohol and food addictions. We're either eating or drinking our way to happiness—or both.

Granted, not everyone has a problem with alcohol. Some people say there are four types of drinkers:

- Light or non

- Weekend-non binge
- Weekend drinkers who get drunk
- Heavy drinkers where every night is party night

The problem with those in the latter two categories may not be the booze, but maladaptive attempts to mask the causal factors.

Addictions and consistent alcohol abuse, in particular, are essentially attempts to escape pain. The nature and causal factors of this pain and the scale of dependency will vary in specifics and severity from person to person.

We all suffer painful experiences—but not everyone has learned to cope in a way that promotes, not depletes emotional, mental, physical and spiritual well-being, health and happiness.

Instead, too often developing and becoming dependent on unhealthy coping techniques becomes the norm—a norm that creates even more problems.

Fortunately, developing more positive ways of coping with life's inevitable ups and downs is not only possible but even enjoyable.

Changing your habits, even very deeply entrenched ones is a learned skill—and you'll find plenty of teachers when you go in search of answers.

Don't wait to hit rock bottom before you do something about your drinking or whatever's going on in your life that causes you to drink too much.

Start now. You can, and you will control your drinking. You don't always need to check in to rehab or pay mega dollars to sit on a psychologist's couch. It's totally fine if that turns out to be your sobriety solution, in full or in part.

The trouble with the 'disempowered' and 'disease' model of addiction, is that a great number of people can lead you to believe that controlling alcohol is completely beyond your reach.

Being told that if you drink too much, you have a disease, an incurable one at that, is neither helpful, truthful, nor empowering—even if it does feel better to know that it's not your fault that you drink too much.

We'll discuss the escalating rise of the disease model of addiction later in this book, but let's look at how some of the pros define addiction and substances abuse—what they focus on and what they miss.

The Maladaptive Pattern of Relying on Alcohol

Psychologists, psychiatrists, and many other addiction specialists predominantly focus on addiction as being a mental disorder, rather than an attempt to self-medicate or anaesthetise ones way through life. Very often a person's personal history of trauma, bullying or societal factors which aid, abet and accelerate their drinking are ignored.

The primary source used to classify problem drinking is provided by the American Psychiatric Association and their Diagnostic and Statistical Manual of Mental Disorders known as the DSM

Over-consuming alcohol is a disease we're told. A disorder of the mind, or an inherited genetic defect. DSM followers turn a blind eye to the fact that alcohol is a self-prescribed, self-served, legalised drug of choice turned to by many as their stress, anxiety, depression, trauma or grief-numbing cure.

Granted, not a particularly robust one, but perhaps, not the 'only-able- to-be-cured-by-medical-professionals' illness we have been led to believe.

"There's an enormous sense of self-medication.... The

fastest thing you can do at the cutting board is open a bottle of wine, pour yourself a glass. It's faster than going to your doctor to say 'I'm suffering from burnout,' it's faster than going to a yoga class and relaxing in a different way," says Dowsett-Johnston.

Even though Johnston knew she was getting into trouble with her drinking she says, "It took two family members and a sweetheart who confronted me, and luckily I took a sledge-hammer and went to rehab and I'm in my 10th year of sobriety."

As you'll discover later in this chapter, with the passing of time alcohol has shifted from being viewed as a problem of faulty, or maladaptive behaviour, to one of disease.

This has opened the route to funding, and the creation of profitable business lines by drug companies scrambling to cure the 'disease' (or what I call the dis-ease) created by the world's most popular and legalised drug.

As a result, they have created a range of pharmaceuticals and manufactured drugs promising the ultimate (and prof-itable) cure. I recently heard they are trying to create an alcohol vaccine. Really? When did loving alcohol too much, or using it as an upper or a sedative, equate with Swine Flu, Chicken Pox, or Aids for that matter?

What if the ultimate cure lies in your own hands—a more mindful, holistic and therapeutic approach to how much you drink and why.

We're told loving alcohol too much is something we can't cure ourselves—that total abstinence is the only remedy. In my professional and personal experience, very often people choose to quit alcohol for good because they're just so over it.

Once alcohol is unmasked for the troublemaker it is, like a shitty lover, people choose never to go back. Whether it's fear of the havoc booze creates, or love—the joy and bliss they discover in their new partnership with life being alcohol-free—people who choose abstinence know life is better, way better, sober.

"You know, I never thought I'd never drink. I loved it, but going sober has forced me to face up to who I really am. I don't always have to be the life of the party. I can just leave and it's okay. So, I've realised I'm a lot more serious than I pretended to be," said the 36-year-old Hayley Holt, former ballroom dancing queen, snowboarding legend and TV star, and the former girlfriend of ex-All Black Captain, Richie McCaw, once said.

So serious in fact in 2017 she turned her set her sober sights high and turned her focus toward Parliament and campaigned in the electorate held by former Prime Minister, Sir John Key, on behalf of The Green Party.

Actor Colin Farrell also testifies that once problem drinking is kicked not only is life infinitely better—*you* are better.

"I have yet to meet a person whose sobriety has made their life worse. I have yet to. But I am open to it. If you find someone please get in touch with me because I would love to have a chat with them and ask them a couple of questions. I have yet to meet a person whose sobriety didn't make a better father, a better friend..."

Kristin Davis, most famous for her role as Charlotte York Goldenblatt in *Sex and the City*, has been alcohol-free since 1987. "Sometimes it would be nice to just have some red wine with dinner, but it's not worth the risk. I have a great life, a great situation. Why would I want risk self-destructive behaviour?"

What do these people and others have in common? Their drinking was a problem—until it wasn't.

The chances are that you don't need a book and checklists

to tell you that you have a problem, but just in case you're amongst the group of people who truly don't know how out of hand your drinking is getting you may be interested to learn what the American Psychiatric Association (APA) classifies as problematic.

What is Problem Drinking?

Regardless of whether you side with alcohol being or not being a disease, the APA classifications of problem drinking include:

- Tolerance and the never decreasing requirement for more
- Withdrawal symptoms when you can't get your fix
- Difficulty in giving up
- Persistent physical, psychological, social, mental and emotional problems that are likely to have been caused or exacerbated by your alcohol

The more symptoms you have, the more urgent the need for change.

Mmmm, using this definition, it would appear 85 percent of the drinking population has a problem. Remember this when people try to shame you for not drinking with taunts such as, "Do you have a problem?" No, my friend, they have the problem.

Addiction (termed substance dependence by the American Psychiatric Association—APA) was once defined as, "a maladaptive pattern of substance use leading to clinically significant impairment or distress."

This maladaptive pattern manifests by three (or more) of

the following, occurring any time in the same 12-month period, say the APA:

1. Tolerance, as defined by either of the following: (a) A need for markedly increased amounts of the substance to achieve intoxication or the desired effect or (b) Markedly diminished effect with continued use of the same amount of the substance.

2. Withdrawal, as manifested by either of the following:

(a) The characteristic withdrawal syndrome for the substance, or

(b) The same (or closely related) substance is taken to relieve or avoid withdrawal symptoms.

3. The substance is often taken in larger amounts or over a longer period than intended.

4. There is a persistent desire or unsuccessful efforts to cut down or control substance use.

5. A great deal of time is spent in activities necessary to obtain the substance, use the substance, or recover from its effects.

6. Important social, occupational, or recreational activities are given up or reduced because of substance use.

7. The substance use is continued despite knowledge of having a persistent physical or psychological problem that is likely to have been caused or exacerbated by the substance (for example, current cocaine use despite recognition of cocaine-induced depression or continued drinking despite recognition that an ulcer was made worse by alcohol consumption).

"We just liked to have a good time."

CAN you tick-off three or more of the above? I bet you never thought of yourself as being maladaptive. As psychologist and founder of *Soberly*, a movement dedicated to supporting sober warriors, Libby Wallace writes,

"I remember a lecture I went to for one of my psychology papers, around 9 years ago, and the lecturer stood at the front and did a 'drinking quiz' similar to the Ministry of Health one to find out whether or not you have a drinking problem. About 60 out of the 100 students put their hands up to say that they had rated themselves with a score that effectively meant they were an alcoholic. After discussing with a few friends after, and in the tutorial later, we thought it was funny and that because we were students, it didn't relate to us, we just liked to have a good time."

Alcohol Use Disorder & The Disease of Alcohol

In 2000 the DSM-IV criteria for substance dependence included several specifiers, one of which outlines whether substance dependence is accompanied by physiological dependence (evidence of tolerance or withdrawal) or without physiological dependence (no evidence of tolerance or withdrawal).

In addition, remission categories are classified into four subtypes: (1) full, (2) early partial, (3) sustained, and (4) sustained partial; on the basis of whether any of the criteria for abuse or dependence have been met and over what time frame.

The remission category can also be used for patients receiving agonist therapy (such as methadone maintenance or drugs designed to control alcohol dependence) or for those living in a controlled, drug-free environment.

This definition was altered in the 5th edition of the DSM.

As compared to DSM-IV, the DSM-5's chapter on addictions was changed from "Substance-Related Disorders" to "Substance-Related and Addictive Disorders" to reflect developing understandings regarding addictions.

The DSM-5 specifically lists nine types of substance addictions within this category (alcohol; caffeine; cannabis; hallucinogens; inhalants; opioids; sedatives, hypnotics, and anxiolytics; stimulants; and tobacco).

These disorders are presented in separate sections, but they are not fully distinct because all drugs taken in excess activate the brain's reward circuitry, and their co-occurrence is common.

Problem drinking that becomes severe is given the medical diagnosis of "alcohol use disorder" or AUD in the DSM-V and is defined in the DSM-5 as a chronic relapsing brain disease characterised by compulsive alcohol use, loss of control over alcohol intake, and a negative emotional state when not using. An estimated 16 million people in the United States have AUD. Approximately 6.2 percent or 15.1 million adults in the United States ages 18 and older had AUD in 2015. This includes 9.8 million men and 5.3 million women. Adolescents can be diagnosed with AUD as well, and in 2015, an estimated 623,000 adolescents ages 12–17 had AUD.

To be diagnosed with AUD, individuals must meet certain criteria outlined in the Diagnostic and Statistical Manual of Mental Disorders (DSM). Under DSM–5, the current version of the DSM, anyone meeting **any two of the 11 criteria during the same 12-month period receives a diagnosis of AUD.**The severity of AUD—mild, moderate, or severe—is based on the number of criteria met.

How Do You Measure Up?

To assess whether you or loved one may have AUD, here are some questions to ask. In the past year, have you:

- Had times when you ended up drinking more, or longer than you intended?
- More than once wanted to cut down or stop drinking, or tried to, but couldn't?
- Spent a lot of time drinking? Or being sick or getting over the after effects?
- Experienced craving—a strong need, or urge, to drink?
- Found that drinking—or being sick from drinking —often interfered with taking care of your home or family? Or caused job troubles? Or school problems?
- Continued to drink even though it was causing trouble with your family or friends?
- Given up or cut back on activities that were important or interesting to you, or gave you pleasure, in order to drink?
- More than once gotten into situations while or after drinking that increased your chances of getting hurt (such as driving, swimming, using machinery, walking in a dangerous area, or having unsafe sex)?
- Continued to drink even though it was making you feel depressed or anxious or adding to another health problem? Or after having had a memory blackout?
- Had to drink much more than you once did to get the effect you want? Or found that your usual

number of drinks had much less effect than
before?
- Found that when the effects of alcohol were
wearing off, you had withdrawal symptoms, such
as trouble sleeping, shakiness, irritability, anxiety,
depression, restlessness, nausea, or sweating? Or
sensed things that were not there?

**REMEMBER that meeting any two of the 11 criteria during
the same 12-month period means you receive a diagnosis
of AUD.**

IF YOU HAVE any of these symptoms, your drinking may
already be a cause for concern. The more symptoms you
have, the more urgent the need for change," say profession-
als. But you know this already—or you wouldn't be reading
this book.

Remember, there is no shame in admitting you have a
problem. You're in good, or is that poor company? You
decide. The true tragedy is not the problem, but not seeking
help.

Like cocaine and heroin, shopping for things we don't
need or eating sweet sugary food is addictive and satisfies our
brain's craving for dopamine until we get our next fix.

Marketing moguls have known this for a long time and
target people indiscriminately. Everywhere you look you're
bombarded with ads about alcohol and sugar fixes that will
cure our blues and make us supposedly happier and
healthier.

Even the stuff dangled as healthier often has something to

hide. Loaded with essential nutrients, natural flavours? Or concealing more than double your daily sugar requirement.

It's time to get wise!

Forget about waiting for law changes, forget about lobbying governments for more enlightened regulations. Take back your power. Open your eyes. It's not easy to change but you can begin by asking yourself more empowering questions, such as:

- Do I really need that fix?
- Will it impact on my wellbeing? How?
- How does alcohol work? Can I find a healthier, cheaper, more effective way to feel better?

The answers may prove illuminating. You may discover, as I have, that a swim in the ocean, a soak in the local hot mineral pools, a night at the movies, a massage, twenty-minutes mediation, or diverting the money I'm saving by not drinking booze for treats like pedicures, delivers a far faster, friendlier fix.

7

WOUNDED WARRIORS

If you're struggling with alcohol abuse or you're using booze to self-medicate, this doesn't necessarily make you an alcoholic—this doesn't mean you have a disorder or an incurable disease.

Self-medicating or anaesthetising yourself with booze doesn't make you hopeless. But it does create an exponential increase that unless you become aware of how much you drink, why you drink and learn how to take back control, you'll continue to over-drink.

A great many people drink alcohol to mask or numb the symptoms of their wounds.

No one escapes walking in this world without some degree of hurt. For many people this hurt is profoundly deep.

The first cuts, experts (and songwriters) say are the deepest—very often these wounds are inflicted during childhood.

Tragically, what should be a happy time of innocence is one of incalculable pain. Incest, rape, physical abuse, emotional neglect—and many more horrid crimes, including murder, are often committed under the influence of alcohol.

Our local tavern, a sports and gambling bar, proudly tells patrons that they can bring their families, yet some 20 metres or so down the road a community noticeboard warns, "Kids are safer when you are sober. Ease up on the drink."

Tragically, it's a message that falls on far too many ears too deaf to hear, eyes too blind, and minds too inebriated to see the truth about alcohol.

Almost no-one escapes the toll of alcohol. Neither money, nor affluence, nor sobriety, nor age escapes its wrath. As I share in the opening of this book, my grandmother was four, and her brother aged six, and were outside the pub when their alcoholic father got into a drunken-brawl and murdered a man. Molly and her brother were forced apart—her brother was adopted and my grandmother spent her childhood being bounced out of foster homes. They never saw each other, or their parents, again.

Walking wounded? You bet. My grandmother spent her life seeking comfort from alcohol, even a stint in rehab couldn't dislodge the habit. Her brother, in adulthood, took his life.

Neither of them was ever offered help to heal the wounds of their past.

In *The Biology of Desire: why addiction is not a disease*, Marc Lewis shares the following testimony from an addiction counsellor and former alcoholic,

"I have had a long hard look inside about how I feel personally about addiction. I do not feel that I have or had a disease. I see my past drinking as a behavioural problem, a learned response to dealing (or not dealing) with emotional pain and stress. Once I achieved the excavating of my wounds I no longer lived with the same anxiety or sense of dread/guilt and shame."

Personally, I have always been troubled by the preference

of mainstream psychology to categorise and pathologize unwellness without delving deeper into its origins.

Instead, wounds are plastered over—seemly *cured* by a steady diet of pills and prescriptions. It was refreshing to read Lewis's book and this account. I encourage you to purchase a copy of his book. It's a brilliant exposé on the truth of addiction and the road to recovery.

Yes, I am overjoyed to say, times are slowly changing. *Slowly.* Unwellness is still a multi-billion dollar industry—there are powerful incentives to keep people dependent on the promise that the latest drug will cure.

Yet there is also an explosion of interest in alternative approaches to health and well-being and with it, the treatment of addiction. Three modern-day factors appear to herald the call for change:

- The escalating epidemic of depression, stress, anxiety and addiction
- The failure of the pharmaceutical industry to come up with sustainable solutions—let alone side-effect-free cures
- A flurry of reputable scientific studies validating the impact of therapies, once devalued and demoted as 'alternative'.

Transcendental meditation, prayer, massage, diet and a wide array of healing modalities, including energy healing, are on the ascent. Science it seems, has finally validated what many ancient cultures have always known—mind, body, spirit and environment are interconnected.

People are waking to the real reasons they drink.

As Legendary rock star Alice Cooper said in an interview,

"I didn't realise that I was an alcoholic until I realised that alcohol was not for fun anymore. It was medicine."

You may, Cooper and others, may identify with the label 'alcoholic.' You may find it empowers you, like finally being given a diagnosis that explains the symptoms of illness that has made you sick for so long.

"I feel better now that I know what it is," so many people say when told that what ails them has a name. But labels can be limiting. Labels can pathologies, categorise, and demoralise. What purpose does it serve to be labeled an alcoholic? What solution does it bring? Perhaps it helps fuel your will. Fantastic. But it just seems like a negative affirmation that feels bad.

Why not say, as I do when offered alcohol, "I don't drink." When people ask, "why not?" I smile and say, "I like it too much."

Rather than spend time on carefully manicured labels consider diving deeper and bringing to light the wounds or triggers that drive you to drink. Consider exorcizing the trauma that has severed your growth, stolen your childhood, blocked your joy and kept you stuck in a cycle of abuse.

Seek help.

- Seek help to heal the wounds of the past
- Seek help to free you from a toxic relationship
- Seek help to liberate you from untenable job stress
- Seek help from whatever or whoever causes you to over-drink.

Perhaps you don't drink to plaster over traumatic wounds. Perhaps your drinking habit is your quick-fix strategy to take the sharp edge off living in this world.

Whatever your reasons, whatever your motivations, whatever has attracted you to this book, it's my sincerest hope that you find encouragement, help, and healing in the pages that follow.

I'd like to encourage you to view this book as Home Rehab—your in-house holistic addiction recovery centre.

Instead of forking out thousands of dollars to be treated by some of the world's most esteemed addiction specialists you'll find some of the best of the best in the pages that follow including:

- A diet of knowledge and education
- The latest developments in mind and body science, including neurotheology, neuroesthetics, psychotherapy and more
- Mind, body, and soul therapies—including energy psychology and holistic healing—including meditation

The Path to Sobriety

I promise to break down the path to sobriety in ways you can easily understand and apply to your own life.

Knowledge is power. Ultimately long-term success in winning the war on alcohol can be explained through medical science and psychology— and marketing...how the booze barons encourage you to act against your best interests.

Understanding alcohol from all angles will offer substantive reasons for why it works.

Importantly, what I'd love you to take away from reading this book is that there is no one path to sobriety. You may or may not be able to go it alone, you may need help, you may need therapy, but regardless of the approach you take, controlling alcohol is a long-term lifestyle change.

Very often, as I've said, it may mean spotlighting and healing the wounds of your past.

Comedian and former addict Russel Brand shares his story of childhood sexual abuse in his book *Recovery: Freedom From Our Addictions.* In his book he reinterprets The Twelve Step recovery process and champions the call for abstinence.

Similarly, Duff McKagan, the former bass guitarist of Guns N' Roses and one of the world's greatest rock musicians, shares how he used alcohol to self-medicate his agonising anxiety. The origin of his pain he says, stemmed from being asked to lie to his mother about his father's affairs, their subsequent divorce and his father's own heavy drinking.

McKagan devised his own program of anxiety treatment and alcohol recovery. Read the inspiring story of a man who partied so hard he nearly died, in his book *It's so Easy and Other Lies.*

Anne Dowsett Johnson, a journalist and self-described recovering alcoholic, and the daughter of an alcoholic herself, urges us all to wake up to the wilful blindness to the damages of drinking in our culture, and explores disturbing trends and false promises peddled by alcohol barons in her book *Drink: The Intimate Relationship Between Women and Alcohol.* For Dowsett, medical intervention through prescribed antidepressants played an instrumental role in her recovery.

AA's 12-step approach didn't work for stressed entrepreneur Russ Parry. But years of therapy, couple counselling , renewing his faith and a program of recovery offered by his church did—alongside changing his relationship to work. He shares his journey to abstinence in his book, *The Sober Entrepreneur.*

These are just some of the many people and books I have

come to admire as I embarked on my own journey to understand why I drank so much and why I couldn't stop.

For these people, sharing their stories was part of their healing process—that and the desire to pay-it-forward. In my book, E*mploy Yourself* from my bestselling *Mid-Life Career Rescue* series, I share how health coach Sheree Clark numbed her job blues by over-drinking until she realised booze was never going to be a long-term sustainable solution.

She sold her business and created a new career as a healthy living coach. She still enjoys a drink—but says since her career change that she couldn't be happier or healthier.

As author and filmmaker Michael Moore said, "I want us all to face our fears and stop behaving like our goal in life is merely to survive. Surviving is for game show contestants stranded in the jungle or on a desert island. You are not stranded. Use your power. You deserve better."

I took these words to heart many years ago. Anxiety and depression run in my family—as does a tendency to place a stop-cap on dreams. As you've read, my grandmother grew up in foster care, plagued by the shame of her family secret— her father was murdered a man. It doesn't matter that he was drunk, that he only meant to land a punch. Murder is murder, right? At least it is to those quick to judge.

I'm sure that Molly's painful upbringing had an impact on how much she drank. She was such a beautiful women with so much truly tragic trauma, including the death of her first child—a much-longed for son who arrived into the world still-born.

My grandmother's upbringing also impacted my mother and her sister. My mom told me that she couldn't recall ever coming home from school without finding her mother in bed. My grandmother's emotional distance and attempts to numb her pain, in turn, impacted my mom's ability to give me the love I craved as a child.

My dad suffered the trauma of emotional neglect too. He was dumped in a boarding school when he was only four—supposedly for his highest good. He never knew his father, and only found out when he was in his 70s that he had a sister. Growing up, he never experienced a hug or knew true affection.

I understand now why, growing up, I, nor my siblings were ever hugged. We still don't. Hugging feels awkward, stiff, painful—foreign.

Like Amy Winehouse and so many others with wounded childhoods, early traumas can leave permanent scars that alcohol and other drugs appear to smooth.

Writing this book has awakened many painful memories, I found myself grieving for the feeling of belonging I never felt. But writing and time has healed these memories too—knowledge, truth, love and acceptance does that.

I've worked hard to overcome the wounds of my child-hood—my adulthood too.

You should, too. Your past doesn't need to stop you.

"A lot of people feel like they're victims in life, and they'll often point to past events, perhaps growing up with an abusive parent or in a dysfunctional family," writes Rhonda Byrne in *The Secret*.

"Most psychologists believe that about 85 percent of families are dysfunctional, so all of a sudden you're not so unique. My parents were alcoholics. My dad abused me. My mother divorced him when I was six... I mean, that's almost everybody's story in some form or not," she says.

The author of the *Chicken Soup For The Soul* series, Jack Canfield, also speaks to this point: "The real question is, what are you going to do now? What do you choose now? Because you can either keep focusing on that, or you can focus on what you want. And when people start focusing on what they want, what they don't want falls away, and what they want expands, and the other part disappears."

In hindsight, you will see your life experiences as a gift. As Isabel Allende once said, "Without my unhappy childhood and dysfunctional family, what would I have to write about?"

I channel my life experiences into my books. I pay it forward and share how I learned to empower my mind, body, and soul. I studied Buddhist philosophy. I learned Transcendental and mindfulness meditation—and praise the life-altering magic of this beautiful tool as often as I can.

Something, fashion designer, Stellar McCartney has also done recently, when in a 2018 article she revealed how in her twenties she turned to meditation after her mother's death. "Transcendental Meditation keeps me sane," McCartney says.

At the time of writing she is 46, and wants everyone to have the chance to reap the same benefits, whether they have a raw emotional need for TM, like she did, or not. Which is why, despite her preference to keep her private life away from the spotlight, she gave her first interview on meditation.

Reading her account, and those of others, fortifies my own spiritual and wellbeing practices. As does reading self-empowerment and personal development books.

When I was struggling with my own anxiety and depression I devoured nearly every self-help book on the planet—and beyond. I went to healers and sought counselling.

I trained to be a hypnotherapist, counsellor, and therapist, and gained other therapeutic skills. I continue to pass on the knowledge I've learned to my clients and readers like you to help empower us all to live our best lives. It's a large part of the motivation behind sharing so much of my own personal story and vulnerabilities in *Your Beautiful Mind*. This is me 'unplugged.'

Every day I fight for my dreams.

We all enter this life, and leave it, with different challenges. Different parents, siblings, life experiences. The pain of your past doesn't need to define you. If you are prepared to be honest and vulnerable and to do the graft, you know what you need to do to empower your life and your work.

Throughout this book we'll explore a diverse range of strategies to help you either ease up on the drink or ditch it entirely. For some people, when they lose the triggers that drive their craving, control comes easily.

For others, alcohol is a serious and dangerously addictive substance—they come to accept that they just can't handle it.

Whatever camp you're in, you are the expert in your own life. You are not powerless to make a change for the better. Empowering yourself is the biggest, most vital, most life-affirming skill of all.

As former addict and leading neuroscientist Marc Lewis writes in this book, *The Biology of Desire: why addiction is not a disease,* alcoholism and addiction "can spring up in anyone's backyard. It attacks our politicians, our entertainers, our relatives, and often ourselves. It's become ubiquitous, expectable, like air pollution and cancer."

Shaming, blaming and naming is not the cure, compassion understanding, and living life on your terms is.

As Lewis also notes, "Many experts highlight the value of empowerment for overcoming addiction. In fact, most former addicts claim that empowerment, not powerlessness, was essential to them, especially in the latter stages of their recovery. Sensitivity to the meaning of empowerment in recovery may be greatest for those who've been disempowered in their social world, including women, minorities, the poor, and those with devastating family histories."

Abusing alcohol is not a disease. It's a coping strategy—one, before reading this book, you may not have been aware of.

As you read this book, you'll reclaim your power and decide whether alcohol has anything positive to contribute to your life at all, or whether you'd be better off putting your money, your energy, your time, your happiness and your health into something, or someone, who's a less abusive lover. Yes, you will decide—it's that simple, and at times, that difficult.

Throughout *Your Beautiful Mind: Control Alcohol,* we'll explore ways to heal the past and exorcize unhelpful emotions that keep you stuck in a cycle of destructive feelings.

As Candace Pert writes in, *Everything You Need to Know to Feel Go(o)d,* "Buried, painful emotions from the past make up what some psychologists and healers call a person's 'core emotional trauma'.

"The point of therapy—including bodywork, some kinds of chiropractic, and energy medicine—is to gently bring that wound to gradual awareness so it can be re-experienced and understood.

"Only then is choice possible, a faculty of your frontal cortex, allowing you to reintegrate any disowned parts of yourself; let go of old traumatic patterns, and become healed, or whole."

Let's take a deeper dive into how to control alcohol before it seizes the throttle and controls you.

DID YOU ENJOY THIS EXCERPT?

.   .   .

YOUR BEAUTIFUL MIND: Control Alcohol and Love Life More: Discover Freedom, Find Happiness & Change Your Life

For readers who sincerely want to stop or rescue their drinking, but struggle to quit the drink habit, this book will pave the way.

Available in print and eBook from all good online bookstores.

COPYRIGHT

The intent of the author is only to offer information of a general nature to help you in your quest for emotional, physical, and spiritual well-being.

Any use of information in this book is at the reader's discretion and risk. Neither the author nor the publisher can be held responsible for any loss, claim or damage arising from the use or misuse of the suggestions made, the failure to take medical advice or for any material on third-party websites.

ISBN PRINT: 978-1-99-105401-2
  ISBN EBOOK: 978-1-99-105400-5

First Edition